GASTRITIS NUTRITION FOR BEGINNERS

Essential Nutrition Plans, Recipes, Dietary Guidelines, And Holistic Approaches To Alleviate Gastritis Discomfort, Restore Digestive Balance And Promote Gut Health

DR. JACE ZAYDEN

Table of Contents

DISCLAIMER

The information provided in the book is intended for general informational purposes only. The content of this book should not be considered a substitute for professional medical advice, diagnosis, or treatment.

Readers are advised to consult with a qualified healthcare professional for medical advice tailored to their individual circumstances.

The author has made every effort to ensure that the information in this book is accurate and up-to-date at the time of publication. However, medical knowledge is constantly evolving, and new research may emerge that could impact the information presented. The author disclaims any responsibility for any adverse effects or consequences resulting from the use of the information provided in this book.

References or mentions of individuals, products, websites, organizations, or other names within this book are for informational purposes only and do not constitute an endorsement. The author has no affiliations with, and makes no endorsements of, any third-party entities mentioned. Readers are encouraged to conduct their own research and exercise their judgment when considering any external resources or recommendations.

The author and the publisher shall have neither liability nor responsibility to any person or entity with respect to any loss, damage, or injury caused or alleged to be caused directly or indirectly by the information contained in this book. Any reliance on the information within this book is at the reader's own risk.

By reading this book, the reader acknowledges and agrees to the terms of this disclaimer. If the reader does not agree with these terms, they should not use the information provided in this book.

ABOUT THIS BOOK

This book "Gastritis Nutrition" is an indispensable resource for those afflicted with gastritis, as it provides a thorough compilation of medical knowledge and pragmatic dietary recommendations. The introductory segment establishes a fundamental comprehension of the intricacies of gastritis, thereby equipping the reader with the necessary knowledge to scrutinize its causes, symptoms, and diagnostic methodologies. Through an exploration of the diverse classifications of gastritis, this book empowers readers to comprehend the intricacies of this gastrointestinal ailment, thereby promoting a more knowledgeable strategy towards its treatment.

An essential element of this book is its examination of the complex correlation that exists between nutrition and gastritis. The dietary recommendations presented offer individuals a systematic approach to managing their culinary selections, while the specific foods that are permitted and prohibited provide pragmatic, implementable guidance. By incorporating meal planning strategies that are customized to address gastritis, one can not only simplify the process of incorporating these strategies but also guarantee a well-rounded and nourishing approach to daily nutrition. The inclusion of nutritional supplements and discussions on lifestyle modifications serve to augment the reader's repertoire of strategies for efficiently managing gastritis.

In addition to discussing dietary considerations, the book provides hydration advice, thereby presenting a comprehensive approach to preserving optimal gastrointestinal health. The incorporation of cooking techniques and recipes that are compatible with gastritis accommodates individuals who prioritize both taste and nutritional value. Furthermore, this book explores the intricate relationship between stress and gastritis, offering readers pragmatic strategies to effectively cope with stress.

This book's concluding chapters provide crucial advice and considerations, with an emphasis on the importance of seeking guidance from a healthcare professional. By customizing the information to suit the needs of specific health conditions, this book guarantees inclusiveness by acknowledging the distinct obstacles encountered by particular populations. Fundamentally, "Gastritis Nutrition" serves as an indispensable manual that not only imparts knowledge but also enables readers to adopt proactive measures in order to effectively manage and alleviate the detrimental effects of gastritis on their general health.

CHAPTER ONE

Introduction

Gastritis, a prevalent gastrointestinal disorder, has life-altering consequences for dietary preferences and the daily lives of millions of people around the globe. A critical factor in the management of gastritis is nutrition, as specific foods have the potential to either mitigate or worsen symptoms. This article examines the correlation between nutrition and gastritis, encompassing its classification, causes, symptoms, and diagnosis.

Comprehension Of Gastritis

Gastritis is an acute or chronic inflammation of the mucosal membrane of the stomach. Composed of cells that produce mucus, the stomach lining safeguards the organ against the corrosive impacts of digestive acids. Inflammation of this lining may result in pain, discomfort, and additional digestive complications.

A multitude of factors are implicated in the pathogenesis of gastritis. Frequent triggers include Helicobacter pylori (H. pylori) infection, prolonged nonsteroidal anti-inflammatory drug (NSAID) use, excessive alcohol consumption, and autoimmune diseases. Additionally, specific infections and stress can contribute to gastritis.

The capacity of the stomach to produce vital digestive enzymes is impaired by the inflammatory process in gastritis, which can also impede the absorption of vital nutrients. Consequently, individuals afflicted with gastritis may encounter deficiencies in essential nutrients; thus, dietary decisions assume a pivotal role in the management of the ailment.

Aetiology Of Gastritis

It is critical to comprehend the etiology of gastritis in order to optimize treatment. As previously stated, H. pylori infection, in which the bacteria cause inflammation by assaulting the gastric lining, is a prevalent factor.

NSAIDs, which are frequently prescribed for the purpose of alleviating pain, have the potential to cause irritation to the gastric mucosa, ultimately culminating in gastritis, particularly when used for extended periods.

Alcohol can also promote inflammation and irritation of the stomach membrane, both of which are factors that can contribute to gastritis. Chronic stress, which is frequently disregarded, can contribute to the onset of gastritis through its impact on the stomach's protective mechanisms and its ability to compromise the immune system.

Gastritis can occasionally manifest as an autoimmune reaction, wherein the stomach lining is erroneously targeted by the body's immune system.

Autoimmune gastritis, an uncommon variant of gastritis, has the potential to induce chronic inflammation and harm to the gastric mucosa.

Diagnosis And Symptoms

It is critical to recognize the symptoms of gastritis in order to intervene promptly. Abdominal pain or discomfort, bloating, nausea, regurgitation, and a sensation of fullness are typical symptoms. Severe cases of gastritis may result in hemorrhage within the gastric mucosa, which may manifest as black or bloody diarrhea and, in certain cases, blood vomiting.

A combination of medical history, physical examination, and diagnostic tests are utilized to ascertain the presence of gastritis. By inserting a flexible tube equipped with a camera into the stomach, endoscopy enables a visual examination of the stomach lining in a direct manner. During endoscopy, biopsies may be obtained to determine the nature and severity of gastritis.

In addition to other diagnostic instruments, blood tests can detect H. pylori infection, bacterial proliferation can be identified through imaging investigations and breath tests. It is of the utmost importance to identify the root cause of gastritis in order to develop an effective treatment regimen that may involve dietary adjustments.

Varieties Of Gastritis

Gastritis is a heterogeneous condition characterized by distinct varieties that arise from different etiological factors. Acute gastritis is a transient inflammation of the gastric mucosa that is frequently precipitated by the consumption of nonsteroidal anti-inflammatory drugs (NSAIDs), excessive alcohol consumption, or infections. This form of gastritis is treatable with medications and lifestyle modifications.

Conversely, chronic gastritis endures for a prolonged duration and has the potential to give rise to more severe complications. As previously stated, autoimmune gastritis is caused by an immune system attack on the stomach membrane.

Prolonged monitoring and management may be necessary to avert complications associated with this form of gastritis.

Erosive gastritis, characterized by erosion of the stomach lining, and non-erosive gastritis, in which inflammation develops without apparent harm, are additional categories of gastritis. Distinguishing symptoms effectively may require specific dietary considerations for each type.

In summary, gastritis is a prevalent gastrointestinal disorder that substantially affects one's day-to-day functioning. In the management of gastritis, nutrition is crucial, as dietary decisions can either mitigate or exacerbate symptoms. A comprehensive comprehension of the etiology, manifestations, and classifications of gastritis is imperative in order to administer efficacious diagnosis and treatment. Adopting a customized dietary regimen that prioritizes stomach-soothing foods while avoiding irritants can make a substantial contribution to the management of gastritis and the enhancement of digestive health as a whole. It is imperative that individuals who suspect they have gastritis or are enduring persistent digestive symptoms seek the guidance of a healthcare professional in order to undergo a thorough assessment and develop an individualized treatment regimen.

Nutrition And Gastritis: An All-Inclusive Analysis

Managing gastroenteritis, which is distinguished by inflammation of the gastric mucosa, can present considerable difficulty. Although medical intervention is of utmost importance, nutrition is equally significant in mitigating symptoms and facilitating the recovery process. An individualized, well-balanced diet can significantly improve the efficacy of gastritis management.

Guidelines Regarding Dietary Gastritis:

1.A balanced diet should be a primary focus for individuals who are afflicted with gastritis. This consists of both micronutrients and macronutrients (carbohydrates, proteins, and lipids; vitamins and minerals, respectively). A comprehensive dietary regimen promotes holistic well-being and facilitates the recovery process.

2. Small, Frequent Meals: To alleviate the strain on the digestive system, it is advisable to consume smaller, more frequent meals rather than three substantial meals. By preventing the stomach from becoming overwhelmed, the likelihood of irritation is diminished.

3. Maintaining proper hydration is essential for all individuals, but particularly so for those who have gastritis. The production of gastric mucus, which creates a protective layer on the stomach membrane, is aided by water. Avoiding carbonated and caffeinated beverages is recommended, as they may worsen symptoms.

4. Adequate Fiber Consumption: Although fiber is vital for maintaining digestive health, an overabundance can cause irritation to an inflamed stomach. Soluble fibers, which are abundant in vegetables, fruits, and cereals, are more digestible and should be prioritized.

1. Lean protein sources, including poultry, fish, tofu, and eggs, offer a viable way to supplement the diet with vital amino acids while minimizing the burden on the digestive system.

2. Complex Carbohydrates: Refined carbohydrates should be avoided in favor of whole cereals such as brown rice, quinoa, and whole wheat bread. These nutrients facilitate the progressive release of energy, thereby inhibiting hyperglycemia.

3. When in doubt, choose fruits that do not contain acids, such as apples, mangoes, and melons. While also being more palatable, they supply vital nutrients and antioxidants.

4. Incorporating non-inflammatory vegetables into one's diet, such as zucchini, beets, and verdant greens, in moderation is advised. They can be cooked or steamed to facilitate digestion.

5. Incorporate healthful lipid sources into your diet, such as nuts, avocados, and olive oil. These lipids have the potential to enhance general health without inducing further irritation to the intestinal mucosa.

CHAPTER TWO

Foods To Prevent When Suffering From Gastritis:

1. Acidic and Spicy Foods: Acidic and spicy foods can exacerbate the symptoms of gastritis. Spicy foods, citrus fruits, tomatoes, and vinegar should be avoided.

2. Fatty foods, particularly those that have been fried or rendered oily, have the potential to impede the digestive process and elevate the susceptibility to irritation. Frozen foods, processed munchies, and fatty cuts of meat should be avoided.

3. Caffeine and alcohol have the potential to induce gastric acid secretion, which may result in heightened irritation. Coffee, tea, alcoholic beverages, and carbonated drinks should be restricted or eliminated.

4. Highly processed and processed foods frequently contain preservatives and additives

that are potentially irritating to the stomach. If feasible, choose unprocessed, whole ingredients.

5. Dairy Products Dairy products may exacerbate the symptoms of gastritis in some individuals. When lactose intolerance is suspected, limiting or avoiding dairy products may be prudent.

Planning Meals To Manage Gastritis: When developing a dietary plan for gastritis, individual preferences and intolerances must be meticulously considered. The following is an example of a diet plan designed to assist people in managing gastritis:

For breakfast,

• Banana slices accompanied by a drizzle of honey over oats.

• Eggs scrambled with broccoli.

• Water or herbal tea.

The midmorning snack consists of:

• Greek yogurt topped with an almond sprinkling.

• Water or an all-fruit smoothie (excluding citrus fruits).

Dish for Lunch:

• A salad consisting of grilled chicken or tofu, cucumber, cherry tomatoes, and a variety of greens.

Serve alongside brown rice or quinoa.

• A lemon and olive oil dressing.

Caffeine chamomile or water.

Snack to Follow:

A portion of apple slices accompanied by a dash of almond butter.

• Water or herbal tea.

Meal: Dinner

• Fish that has been grilled or baked alongside steaming vegetables (carrots, zucchini, and broccoli).

Byway potato or brown rice, please.

• A non-acidic, mild sauce.

Water or ginger tea may be used.

Snack in the evening (if required):

• A portion of fruit that is not citrus in nature, such as a melon or pear.

• Water or tea made with peppermint.

It is advisable for individuals diagnosed with gastritis to customize this regimen in accordance with their particular dietary restrictions and sensitivities. Seeking guidance from a registered dietitian or healthcare professional can offer individualized recommendations for effectively managing gastritis via nutritional means.

 It is of the utmost importance to prioritize symptom relief, healing, and overall well-being when devising meal plans.

Gastritis Nutrition: A Healthy Stomach Nutrient

Gastritis is a pathological state distinguished by inflammation of the gastric mucosa, potentially resulting in malaise and gastrointestinal complications. Appropriate nutrition is essential for the management of gastritis, the promotion of healing, and the prevention of exacerbation of symptoms. Gaining knowledge of the fundamentals of gastritis nutrition can enable individuals to make well-informed dietary decisions that promote improved gastric health.

Supportive Nutritional Supplements For Stomach Healing

The integration of nutritional supplements into a regimen for managing gastritis can offer specific assistance for the restoration of the stomach and the promotion of general health. Although it is crucial to seek guidance from a healthcare professional prior to incorporating supplements into one's regimen, the following are some frequently suggested alternatives:

1. Probiotics: These advantageous bacteria facilitate digestion and decrease inflammation by promoting a healthy balance in the gastrointestinal microbiome. Beneficial forms of supplements, yogurt, and kefir exist.

2. Omega-3 fatty acids, which are anti-inflammatory in nature, are discovered in fatty fish, flaxseeds, and hazelnuts. Consider supplementing with fish oil to improve your consumption and support your gastrointestinal health.

3. Vitamin B12: Gastric ulcer patients may experience challenges in the absorption of B12 from their diet. B12 supplementation can prevent deficiency, which is prevalent in cases of chronic gastritis.

4. Zinc is a vital mineral that promotes wound healing and immune function. Although lean meats, nuts, and seeds are nutritious dietary sources, those with deficiencies may require supplements.

5. Anemia may result from chronic gastritis-induced impairment of iron absorption. While iron supplements may be recommended to treat this deficiency, it is imperative to seek personalized guidance from a healthcare professional.

Lifestyle Modifications: An All-Encompassing Strategy For The Management Of Gastritis

Implementing lifestyle modifications is crucial for the effective management of gastritis. These modifications not only mitigate symptoms but also enhance overall health and wellness. Consider the following modifications to your lifestyle:

1. Management of Stress Prolonged stress can worsen the symptoms of gastritis. Daily routines should include stress-relieving activities such as yoga, meditation, and deep breathing exercises.

2. Consistent physical activity, specifically moderate exercise, facilitates metabolism and enhances blood circulation. It is advisable to seek

guidance from your healthcare provider in order to ascertain appropriate activities that are compatible with your current health condition.

3. Alcohol Moderation and Cessation of Smoking: Excessive alcohol consumption and smoking can exacerbate gastritis. Alcohol restriction and smoking cessation are factors that contribute to improved gastric health.

4. Meal Timing and Portion Control: To alleviate gastric discomfort, it is advisable to consume smaller, more frequent meals dispersed throughout the day. It is vital to avoid consuming large, weighty meals and ingesting late at night in order to prevent irritation.

5. Identifying Trigger Foods: Maintain vigilance regarding the foods that elicit or exacerbate your symptoms. Typical irritants consist of acidic substances, caffeine, and piquant foods. Eliminate these triggers from your diet in order to alleviate discomfort.

CHAPTER THREE

Sufficient Hydration: Quenching Thirsts Without Causing Irritation

Although adequate hydration is critical for general well-being, individuals who have gastritis should exercise caution when selecting their beverages. Adhere to the following hydration guidelines to maintain proper hydration while preventing irritation to the gastrointestinal lining:

1. Plaque water is the optimal option for maintaining hydration without causing gastric irritation. Sip at least eight glasses of wine leisurely throughout the day.

2. Select herbal infusions that do not contain caffeine, such as ginger or chamomile tea. These substances may induce gastric relief and serve as a delightful substitute for simple water.

3. Avoid Irritating Beverages: Carbonated beverages, caffeinated beverages, and acidic fluids should be avoided. These can impede the healing process and worsen the symptoms of gastritis.

4. Beverages at Room Temperature: Eating cold or hot beverages may cause irritation to the gastric mucosa. Choose liquids at ambient temperature to reduce the risk of irritation.

Illustrative Of Gastritis-Friendly Recipes: Satiating And Hypoallergenic

Meals designed to be compatible with gastritis require the use of nutritious ingredients that are also gentle on the stomach. To commence, here is a straightforward recipe:

Rice Bowl with Ginger Chicken: Ingredients:

• 1 cup white rice, cooked

• 1 breast of boneless, skinless chicken, minced and broiled

• 1 tablespoon minced fresh ginger

• 1 cup carrots, stewed

1) Tonne of olive oil

• Pepper and salt to flavor

Means of instruction:

1. Sauté grated ginger in olive oil in a saucepan until aromatic.

2.Cook the minced chicken until it is completely cooked.

3. To taste, season with salt and pepper.

4. Serve alongside steamed vegetables over prepared white rice.

This culinary preparation integrates readily assimilated components such as rice, lean poultry protein, and the calming attributes of ginger.

Cooking Methods For Gastritis: Delicate Stomach-Friendly Techniques

It is critical to select the proper cooking methods when producing dishes that are suitable for individuals with gastritis. Select methodologies that are hypoallergenic and preserve the nutritional integrity of foods:

1. By steaming, nutrients are preserved and foods become more easily digestible. This technique can

be employed to prepare vegetables, fish, poultry, and fish.

2. Poaching: Foods that are poached in bouillon or water remain moist and are easier on the stomach. This complements lean proteins such as fish and poultry.

3. Baking or roasting is a healthful culinary method that improves the flavor of proteins and vegetables while minimizing the use of added fats and preventing gastric irritation.

4. Boiling cereals and vegetables in water is an easy and efficient method of cooking that softens and improves the digestibility of the foods.

5. Lean meats should be grilled, as this method permits superfluous fat to drain away. For enhanced flavor, marinate with mild, stomach-friendly herbs and seasonings.

In summary, the effective management of gastritis via nutrition necessitates a comprehensive strategy that integrates dietary modifications, lifestyle adaptations, and conscientious meal planning. You can promote gastric healing, alleviate symptoms, and improve your overall health by integrating these principles into your daily regimen. It is strongly advised to seek personalized guidance from a healthcare professional regarding your specific condition.

Stress Management And Gastritis

Gastritis, which is an inflammation of the membrane of the stomach, can be exacerbated by a multitude of factors, with tension being a significant contributor. In addition to exerting an influence on mental health, stress can also significantly affect digestive health. Effective stress management is essential for individuals afflicted with gastritis in order to mitigate symptoms and enhance general health.

The secretion of hormones such as cortisol and adrenaline in response to stress can cause disturbances in the regular operation of the digestive system. Within the framework of gastritis, elevated gastric acid production and inflammation can be exacerbated by stress. Consequently, the symptoms of gastritis, including pain, bloating, and discomfort, are exacerbated.

In order to optimize stress management, individuals diagnosed with gastritis may integrate tension-reducing activities into their daily schedule. It has been demonstrated that regular exercise effectively alleviates tension by stimulating the release of endorphins, which are the body's innate mood enhancers. Additionally, practices such as yoga and meditation are advantageous because they reduce tension and soothe the mind.

The function of diet in stress management and gastritis is critical. By incorporating nutrient-dense foods into a balanced diet, one can equip the body with the essential mechanisms to manage stress. Incorporate omega-3-rich foods, such as flaxseeds and salmon, into your diet. These fats have been associated with a reduction in tension.

Furthermore, the consumption of complex carbohydrates, such as those found in whole grains and legumes, has the potential to regulate blood sugar levels, thereby mitigating the occurrence of mood fluctuations that are linked to stress.

It is crucial to identify stressors and, whenever possible, avoid them. This may require establishing boundaries, altering one's lifestyle, and placing self-care as a top priority. Additionally, sufficient sleep is crucial, as sleep deprivation can heighten tension levels and worsen symptoms associated with gastritis. It is essential to establish a regular sleep schedule and create a conducive sleeping environment in order to effectively manage tension and enhance digestive health.

Considerations And Precautions

In the context of managing gastritis, implementing specific dietary and lifestyle modifications that adhere to precautions and considerations can substantially aid in alleviating symptoms and averting the condition's inflammation.

1. Dietary Selections:

AVOID Trigger Foods: Specific foods have the potential to provoke gastritis symptoms by irritating the gastric mucosa. Common triggers include acidic and spicy foods and beverages, caffeine, and alcohol. These substances should be identified and eliminated from the diet of individuals with gastritis.

• Adhere to a Low-Fat Diet: Foods high in fat have the potential to induce gastric acid secretion, which may exacerbate the condition. It is beneficial to select low-fat options and avoid fried and fatty foods.

• Small, Regular Meals: Opting for smaller, more frequent meals instead of large, weighty meals can assist in alleviating gastric discomfort and promoting digestive ease.

2. Sufficient hydration:

One should restrict the consumption of carbonated and caffeinated beverages, as they may stimulate the production of gastric acid. It is recommended to consume water, herbal infusions, and non-caffeinated, non-acidic beverages.

3. Proper Meal Timing:

• It is advisable to refrain from late-night eating, as doing so in close proximity to slumber may induce acid reflux, which can have adverse effects on individuals with gastritis. The last supper of the day should be consumed at least a few hours prior to nighttime.

4. Lifestyle Adjustments:

Quit smoking: The gastrointestinal lining can become irritated by smoking, which can hinder the healing process. It is vital to quit smoking in order to effectively manage gastritis and improve overall health. It is advisable to restrict alcohol consumption as it can worsen the symptoms of gastritis. It is advised to exercise moderation or completely abstain from utilization.

5. Medication Administration:

It is imperative that individuals taking gastritis medications, including proton pump inhibitors and antacids, adhere to the prescribed regimen. Medication self-adjustment and missed doses can impede the healing process.

6. Observation of Symptoms:

It is critical to possess knowledge of one's personal triggers and to diligently observe symptoms. By keeping a food diary, one can discern particular foods or circumstances that exacerbate gastritis. Implementing these precautions and factors into account can substantially aid in the control of gastritis. However, it is imperative that individuals seek personalized guidance from healthcare professionals in regard to their particular condition.

CHAPTER FOUR

Seeking Advice From A Healthcare Professional

Although lifestyle modifications are crucial in the management of gastritis, it is imperative to seek the guidance of a healthcare professional in order to obtain a comprehensive and individualized treatment plan. A variety of healthcare professionals, such as dietitians and gastroenterologists, are capable of providing individualized recommendations based on a patient's medical history and current condition.

1. Medical Assessment:

Gastroscopy, blood tests, and imaging studies are examples of diagnostic procedures that may be performed in order to ascertain the extent and fundamental etiology of gastritis.

• Medication Management: To alleviate symptoms and promote healing, healthcare professionals may prescribe proton pump inhibitors, antibiotics (if bacterial infection is present), and antacids.

2. Dietary Recommendations:

Personalised Nutrition Plans: In accordance with an individual's gastritis type and triggers, dietitians have the ability to develop customised nutrition plans. This may entail the exclusion of particular food items, the inclusion of foods that inhibit inflammation, and the maintenance of adequate nutrient consumption.

• Supplementation: Healthcare practitioners may advise the use of vitamin or mineral supplements to compensate for deficiencies that may arise as a result of gastritis or its therapeutic interventions.

3. The practice of lifestyle counseling:

• Strategies for Stress Management: Healthcare experts are capable of offering counsel regarding efficacious stress management techniques, taking into account the correlation between stress and gastritis.

• Smoking Cessation Programs: Healthcare providers have the capacity to provide assistance and resources to smokers in order to facilitate their cessation.

4. Continuation and Monitoring:

Conducting routine check-ups with healthcare professionals is essential in order to assess progress, make necessary adjustments to treatment plans, and attend to any emergent concerns.

By maintaining a symptom diary and expeditiously documenting any alterations or exacerbations of symptoms, medical professionals are able to implement opportune modifications to the treatment regimen.

5. Emergency Circumstances:

• Urgent Medical Attention: Those who are confronted with severe symptoms, including chronic vomiting, substantial weight loss, or indications of gastrointestinal hemorrhage, ought to seek medical attention without delay.

Seeking guidance from healthcare professional guarantees that individuals afflicted with gastritis are provided with all-encompassing treatment that surpasses the mere management of symptoms. It permits a more comprehensive understanding of the root causes and facilitates the formulation of a holistic treatment strategy.

Gastritis In Populations That Are Special

Gastritis is a condition that impacts people of all ages and demographics; however, the management of this condition may necessitate specific considerations for certain populations.

1. Gastritis in Pediatric Patients:

• Thorough Dietary Planning: Diligent dietary planning may be necessary in pediatric cases due to the nutritional requirements that are specific to their growth and development. It is advisable to seek the advice of a pediatrician or pediatric gastroenterologist regarding suitable dietary options and nutritional supplements.

• Career Communication: Maintaining transparent lines of communication with parents or caregivers is of utmost importance in order to guarantee compliance with treatment regimens, particularly with regard to dietary limitations and medication oversight.

2. During pregnancy, gastroenteritis can occur.

Pregnant women who are experiencing gastritis should seek guidance from an obstetrician or gastroenterologist in order to ascertain the appropriateness of medications for their condition. Medication use and the potential effects of gastritis on the developing fetus must be carefully weighed.

• Nutrient Requirements: It is critical to maintain sufficient nutrient consumption throughout pregnancy. Healthcare personnel possess the ability to offer recommendations regarding a well-balanced diet that not only alleviates the symptoms of gastritis but also fulfills the nutritional requirements of the developing embryo.

3. The elderly demographic:

Concerning medication management, the elderly may be more susceptible to adverse effects. Healthcare providers ought to meticulously deliberate on the selection and dosage of medications in order to effectively manage gastritis while concurrently mitigating potential risks.

• Adaptations to Diet: Dietary modifications may be required in light of various factors, including oral health and challenges with chewing. Nutrient-dense and texture-modified foods might be suggested.

4. Conditions of Health Underlying:

• Comorbidities: The management of gastritis in individuals with underlying health conditions, such as diabetes or autoimmune disorders, may necessitate a multidisciplinary approach that attends to the specific requirements of their overall health.

• Medication Interactions: It is crucial to closely monitor special populations that are prescribed multiple medications for various conditions in order to mitigate the risk of potential drug interactions that may compromise the efficacy of gastritis treatment.

5. Psychosocial Assistance:

• Emotional Well-being: With regard to emotional well-being, special populations may encounter distinct obstacles. It is imperative to integrate mental health considerations into the treatment plan and offer psychosocial support in order to promote holistic wellness.

A customized strategy is imperative when it comes to the management of gastritis in special populations, taking into account their unique requirements, possible complications, and the interplay between gastritis and other health determinants.

It may be imperative to foster collaboration among healthcare professionals hailing from diverse specialties in order to deliver comprehensive treatment for these individuals.

In summary, the management of gastritis necessitates an integrated strategy that incorporates stress reduction, adherence to precautions and considerations, consultation with healthcare experts, and special population considerations.

Through the implementation of a comprehensive approach that considers the emotional, dietary, and physical dimensions of gastritis, individuals have the potential to elevate their overall health and life satisfaction.

Consistent communication with healthcare providers and a dedication to making adjustments to one's lifestyle are essential elements in effectively managing gastritis among populations with diverse characteristics.

Conclusion

In summary, effective gastritis management via dietary modifications is vital for symptom relief and the promotion of digestive health as a whole. A judicious and well-rounded dietary regimen that prioritizes soft, easily digestible foods may effectively alleviate irritation and discomfort experienced by the inflamed gastric mucosa. The healing process is aided by the consumption of anti-inflammatory foods, including fruits, vegetables, whole cereals, and lean proteins.

It is critical to refrain from consuming trigger foods such as those that are fiery, acidic, or fattening in order to effectively manage gastritis and prevent flare-ups and exacerbation of symptoms. In addition, avoiding irritants such as alcohol and caffeine helps to preserve a healthy gastrointestinal environment. Ensuring adequate hydration is critical for optimal digestion and to prevent dehydration, both of which can exacerbate the symptoms of gastritis.

In addition, portion control and the consumption of small, frequent meals throughout the day can alleviate the strain on the digestive system and prevent the production of excessive gastric acid. It is imperative to seek guidance from a registered dietitian or a healthcare professional in order to receive individualized dietary recommendations that are tailored to the particular type and severity of gastritis.

Through the implementation of a conscientious and individualized nutritional strategy, people diagnosed with gastritis can proactively aid in the prevention and management of symptoms, thereby promoting sustained gastrointestinal health. By adopting a way of life that places emphasis on consuming foods that promote digestive health, individuals can regain agency over their gastritis and improve their overall standard of living.

THE END